Hormone Harmony Cookbook

A Guide to Balancing Your Body Naturally

Bryan Wealth

Copyright © [2023] by [Bryan Wealth]

All right reserved. No part of this publication may be reproduced, distributed, transmitted in any form or by any means, including photocopying, recording,or other electronic mechanical methods, without the prior written permission of the publisher, except in the case of brief quotations embodied in critical reviews and certain other noncommercial uses permitted by copyright law.

Table of contents

INTRODUCTION

Maintaining hormonal balance is essential for overall well-being, as hormones play a crucial role in regulating various bodily functions. From mood and energy levels to metabolism and reproductive health, hormones are the chemical messengers that keep our body systems in harmony. However, in today's fast-paced and stressful lifestyles, many individuals struggle with hormonal imbalances, leading to a range of health issues. A comprehensive and informative resource designed to help individuals restore and maintain hormonal equilibrium naturally. This guide offers a collection of delicious, nutrient-dense cookbook crafted to support hormonal health and optimize overall vitality.At its core, the Hormone Harmony cookbook is grounded in the principle that food can be a powerful tool to promote hormonal Balance. The cookbook within the guide are carefully curated to incorporate a diverse array of whole foods, rich in essential nutrients, vitamins, and minerals that influence hormonal regulation positively. By embracing a balanced and nourishing diet, individuals can potentially mitigate the negative effects of hormonal imbalances and foster better health outcomes.This guide aims to educate readers about the impact of various nutrients on hormone production and function. It provides insights into how certain foods can either promote or disrupt hormonal balance, empowering individuals to make informed choices about their diet and lifestyle. By understanding the connections between nutrition and hormones, readers can proactively take charge of their health and work towards achieving greater equilibrium.Whether struggling with conditions like polycystic ovary syndrome (PCOS), thyroid disorders, or simply seeking to optimize overall hormonal well-being, the Hormone Harmony cookbook is a valuable resource. It encourages individuals to embark on a journey towards better health and vitality, using the power of wholesome, delicious, and hormone-supportive cookbook.

CHAPTER ONE

Understanding Hormones and Their Impact

Ductless glands system create hormones, which are chemical messengers.They play a crucial role in regulating various physiological processes and maintaining overall balance within the body. Understanding hormones and their impact is essential to grasp how they influence our health and well-being.

1. Hormone Production: Glands, such as the pituitary, thyroid, adrenal, and reproductive glands, produce hormones in response to specific signals from the nervous system or other hormones. Each hormone has a specific target tissue or organ where it exerts its effects.

2. Regulation and Feedback: Hormone secretion is tightly regulated through feedback mechanisms. When hormone levels reach a certain threshold, the

ductless system reduces or stops production to maintain equilibrium.

3. Types of Hormones: There are several types of hormones, including steroids, peptides, and amino acid-derived hormones. Each type has distinct functions and targets.

4. Impact on Body Functions: Hormones influence a wide range of bodily functions, such as metabolism, growth, reproduction, mood, sleep, and stress response. For example, insulin regulates blood sugar levels, while thyroid hormones control metabolism.

5. Homeostasis: Hormones help maintain homeostasis, which is the body's ability to maintain stable internal conditions despite external changes. They ensure that physiological parameters stay within healthy ranges.

6. Hormonal Disorders: Imbalances in hormone levels can lead to various hormonal disorders, such as diabetes, thyroid disorders, and adrenal insufficiency. These conditions can have significant impacts on health if left untreated.

7. Hormones and Development: During development, hormones play a critical

role in shaping the body and its functions. They are instrumental in puberty, growth, and sexual maturation.

8. External Factors: Hormones can be influenced by external factors like stress, diet, exercise, and environmental toxins. These factors can either disrupt hormonal balance or support overall well-being.

9. Hormone Replacement Therapy: In some cases, hormone imbalances or deficiencies are treated with hormone replacement therapy (HRT). This involves administering hormones to restore proper function and alleviate symptoms.

10. The Menstrual Cycle: Hormones play a pivotal role in the menstrual cycle of females, orchestrating ovulation, menstruation, and pregnancy. Understanding these hormonal fluctuations is crucial for reproductive health.

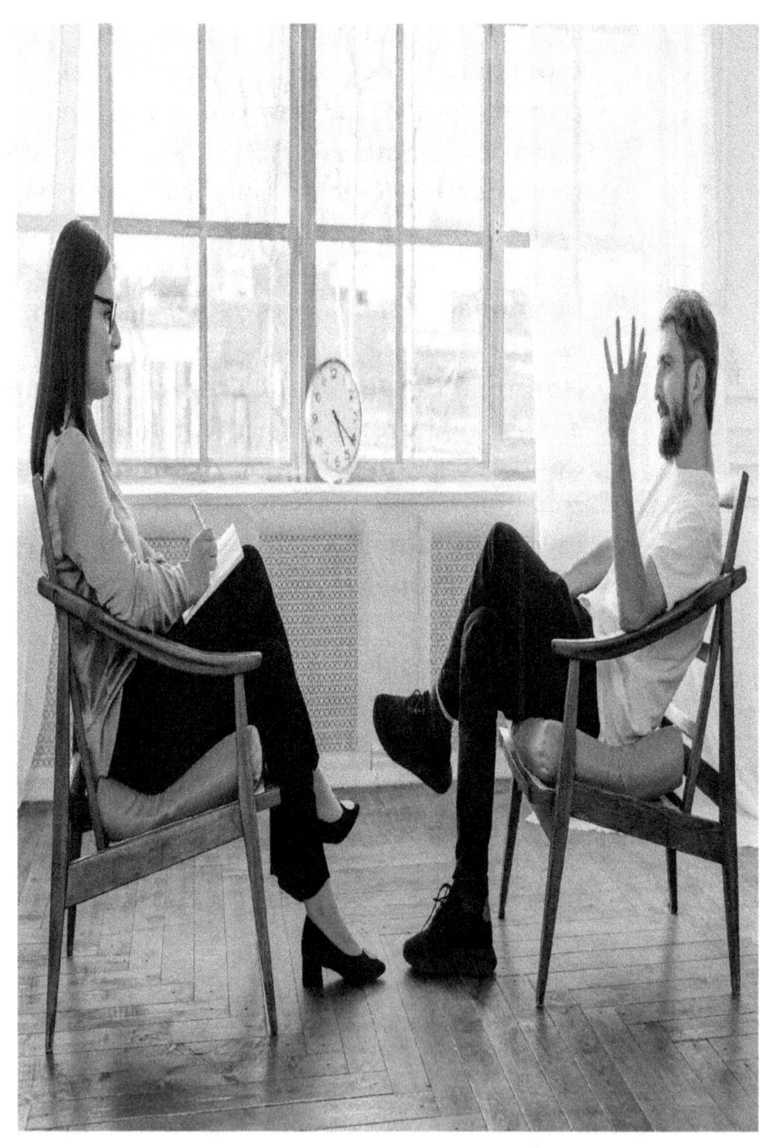

CHAPTER TWO

Balancing Hormones through Nutrition

Nutrient-Rich Foods for Hormone Balance

Nutrient-rich foods that can help support hormone balance include:

1. **Omega-3 Fatty Acids: Found in fatty fish (salmon, mackerel), chia seeds, and flaxseeds, these fats are essential for hormone production and can reduce inflammation.**
2. **Fiber-Rich Foods: Whole grains, fruits, vegetables, and legumes are high in fiber, which aids in hormone regulation by promoting steady blood sugar levels.**
3. **Cruciferous Vegetables: Broccoli, cauliflower, cabbage, and Brussels sprouts contain compounds that support estrogen metabolism and balance.**

4. **Healthy Fats:** Avocados, nuts, and olive oil provide monounsaturated fats that are important for hormone production.

5. **Antioxidant-Rich Foods:** Berries, leafy greens, and colorful fruits and vegetables help combat oxidative stress and promote overall hormonal health.

6. **Probiotic Foods:** Yogurt, kefir, and fermented foods support gut health, which is linked to hormone regulation and balance.

7. **Zinc-Rich Foods:** Foods like pumpkin seeds, oysters, and beans can help maintain healthy testosterone levels.

8. **Vitamin D Sources:** Sunlight exposure, fortified dairy products, and fatty fish contribute to vitamin D intake, which plays a role in hormone synthesis.

By incorporating these nutrient-rich foods into your diet, you can support hormone balance and overall well-being. However, it's essential to maintain a balanced diet and consult a healthcare professional for personalized advice on hormonal health.

Hormone-Supportive Herbs and Spices

Hormone-supportive herbs and spices are natural substances that may help balance hormones and support overall hormonal health. These are some examples and their explanations:

1. Maca root: Maca is known for its adaptogenic properties, which means it can help the body adapt to stress and regulate hormone production. It's often used to support hormonal balance, particularly in women.

2. Ashwagandha: Another powerful adaptogenic herb, ashwagandha, has been traditionally used to reduce stress and support adrenal gland function, which can have a positive impact on hormone levels.

3. Chasteberry (Vitex): Chasteberry has been studied for its potential to help regulate menstrual cycles in women by influencing the production of certain hormones, such as progesterone.

4. Turmeric: The active compound in turmeric, curcumin, has anti-inflammatory properties and may

help support hormone balance by reducing inflammation in the body.

5. Cinnamon: Cinnamon has been linked to improved insulin sensitivity, which can help balance blood sugar levels and support hormone regulation, especially in cases of insulin resistance.

6. Holy basil: Also known as tulsi, holy basil is an adaptogenic herb that can help combat stress, reduce cortisol levels, and support overall hormonal equilibrium.

7. Fenugreek: Fenugreek seeds are rich in compounds that may help regulate blood sugar levels, which in turn can positively impact hormone balance.

8. Rhodiola: Rhodiola is an adaptogenic herb that may help support the adrenal glands and reduce stress, thereby indirectly influencing hormone production and balance.

It's important to note that while these herbs and spices may have hormone-supportive properties, they should not be used as a substitute for medical advice or treatment. Before adding new herbs or supplements to your regimen, always get medical advice, especially if you have underlying health issues or are taking medication.

Plant-Based Protein Sources

Plant-based protein sources are food options derived from plants that provide a significant amount of protein. Some common and nutritious plant-based protein sources include:

1. Legumes: These include beans (black beans, kidney beans, chickpeas), lentils, and peas. They are rich in protein, fiber, and various vitamins and minerals.

2. Nuts and Seeds: Almonds, walnuts, chia seeds, flaxseeds, and pumpkin seeds are excellent sources of protein, healthy fats, and essential nutrients.

3. Grains: Quinoa, brown rice, oats, and whole wheat are grains that offer a good amount of protein and are also rich in fiber and other nutrients.

4. Soy Products: Tofu, tempeh, and edamame are derived from soybeans and are complete protein sources, containing all essential amino acids.

5. Seitan: Made from wheat gluten, seitan is a high-protein meat substitute often used in vegan and vegetarian dishes.

6. Green Vegetables: Spinach, broccoli, kale, and other leafy greens contain

protein along with a host of vitamins and minerals.

7. Plant-Based Protein Powders: Protein powders derived from peas, hemp, rice, or soy can be used as supplements to increase protein intake.

Plant-based protein sources are beneficial as they typically have lower saturated fat content compared to animal-based proteins and are often rich in fiber and antioxidants, promoting overall health and reducing the risk of chronic diseases. Incorporating a variety of these sources into your diet can help you meet your protein needs while following a plant-based or vegetarian lifestyle.

CHAPTER THREE

Breakfast Delights for Hormone Harmony

Energizing Smoothies and Bowls

Here are some energizing smoothies and bowls, along with their explanations:

1. Green Power Smoothie: This smoothie is packed with leafy greens like spinach or kale, along with fruits like banana and pineapple. It provides a good balance of vitamins, minerals, and antioxidants, which can help boost energy levels and promote overall well-being.

2. Berry Blast Smoothie: A mix of berries such as strawberries, blueberries, and raspberries, this smoothie is rich in antioxidants and vitamin C. These nutrients can support your immune system and provide a natural energy boost.

3. Tropical Energy Bowl: A refreshing blend of tropical fruits like mango, papaya, and coconut water, topped with granola and chia seeds. This bowl offers a

combination of carbohydrates and healthy fats that can provide sustained energy throughout the day.

4. Banana Almond Butter Smoothie: Combining the natural sweetness of bananas with the richness of almond butter, this smoothie is a great source of protein and healthy fats, providing long-lasting energy and helping to keep you full.

5. Acai Berry Bowl: Made with acai berries, this bowl is rich in antioxidants and essential nutrients. Topped with fresh fruits, nuts, and seeds, it's a satisfying and energizing option for a nutritious breakfast or snack.

6. Energizing Matcha Smoothie: Matcha green tea powder blended with almond milk, banana, and a touch of honey. Matcha contains caffeine and L-theanine, which can provide a gentle, sustained energy boost without the jitters often associated with coffee.

7. Protein Power Bowl: A blend of protein-rich ingredients like Greek yogurt, hemp seeds, and nut butter, topped with fruits and granola. This bowl can aid in muscle recovery and provide a steady release of energy.

These energizing smoothies and bowls are not only delicious but also packed with nutrients that can help increase vitality and sustain your energy levels throughout the day. They are great options for a healthy and wholesome breakfast or snack. Remember to adjust the ingredients according to your taste preferences and dietary needs. Enjoy!

Wholesome Oatmeal Variations

Here are some wholesome oatmeal variations for a delicious and nutritious breakfast:

1. Classic Apple Cinnamon Oatmeal: Cook oats with water or milk, then add diced apples, a sprinkle of cinnamon, and a drizzle of honey or maple syrup for sweetness.
2. Berry Blast Oatmeal: Mix in your favorite berries (strawberries, blueberries, or raspberries) along with some chia seeds and a dollop of Greek yogurt for added creaminess.
3. Nutty Banana Oatmeal: Slice bananas and add them to your cooked oats. Top with a handful of chopped nuts like almonds or walnuts for a satisfying crunch.
4. Coconut Mango Oatmeal: Stir in diced ripe mangoes and coconut flakes to

create a tropical-inspired oatmeal. Add a splash of coconut milk for a creamy texture.

5. Peanut Butter Chocolate Oatmeal: Mix in a spoonful of natural peanut butter and a dash of cocoa powder to turn your oatmeal into a tasty dessert-like treat.

6. Chai Spice Oatmeal: Infuse your oats with warm chai spices like cinnamon, ginger, and cardamom. Add a touch of honey and a splash of milk for a comforting flavor.

7. Pumpkin Spice Oatmeal: During the fall season, blend in some pumpkin puree, pumpkin spice mix, and a drizzle of maple syrup for a cozy autumn delight.

8. Savory Mediterranean Oatmeal: Try a savory version by adding sautéed vegetables like spinach, cherry tomatoes, and feta cheese to your cooked oats.

9. Almond Joy Oatmeal: Mix in shredded coconut, sliced almonds, and dark chocolate chips to recreate the flavors of the popular candy bar in a healthier way.

10. Green Smoothie Oatmeal: Blend spinach or kale with bananas and milk, then cook your oats in this green smoothie mixture for a nutrient-packed breakfast.

Oatmeal is a versatile base that pairs well with various fruits, nuts, and spices. These wholesome oatmeal variations provide a range of flavors, textures, and nutrients to make your breakfasts enjoyable and nourishing. Whether you prefer a sweet, fruity oatmeal or a savory option, these ideas offer a great way to start your day with a filling and balanced meal. Remember to adjust the ingredients according to your taste and dietary preferences. Enjoy!

Nourishing Breakfast Wraps

Here's a recipe for Nourishing Breakfast Wraps:

Ingredients:

- Whole wheat tortillas or wraps
- Eggs (scrambled or fried)
- Avocado slices
- Baby spinach leaves
- Cherry tomatoes (sliced)
- Feta or cottage cheese (optional)
- Salsa or hot sauce (optional)
- Salt and pepper to taste

Instructions:

1. Cook the scrambled or fried eggs to your liking, and season with salt and pepper.

2. Lay out a whole wheat tortilla or wrap on a flat surface.
3. Place a layer of baby spinach leaves on the tortilla, followed by the cooked eggs.
4. Add avocado slices, cherry tomatoes, and crumbled feta or cottage cheese if desired.
5. Drizzle with salsa or hot sauce for some extra flavor, if you like.
6. The tortilla should be tightly rolled, with the sides folded in as you go to form a wrap.
7. Slice the wrap in half for easier handling, if needed.
8. Serve immediately and enjoy your nourishing breakfast wrap!

Feel free to alter the ingredients to fit your dietary restrictions and taste preferences. Enjoy your delicious and healthy breakfast!

CHAPTER FOUR

Nourishing Lunches for Hormonal Health

Vibrant Salads with Hormone-Balancing Dressings

Vibrant salads with hormone-balancing dressings can be a delicious and nutritious option for lunch. These salads typically contain ingredients that support hormone health and are packed with nutrients. Here are some examples of vibrant salads and hormone-balancing dressings:

1. Green Goddess Salad: A mix of leafy greens, avocado, broccoli, sprouts, and hemp seeds, topped with a hormone-balancing dressing made from tahini, lemon juice, garlic, and a touch of tamari.

2. Rainbow Quinoa Salad: A colorful combination of quinoa, bell peppers, cherry tomatoes, cucumber, and fresh herbs, paired with a dressing containing

olive oil, apple cider vinegar, Dijon mustard, and a sprinkle of flaxseed.

3. Beet and Spinach Salad: Roasted beets, baby spinach, walnuts, and crumbled goat cheese, drizzled with a hormone-balancing dressing made from balsamic vinegar, extra virgin olive oil, and honey.

4. Asian Slaw Salad: Shredded cabbage, carrots, edamame, and sliced almonds, tossed in a hormone-balancing dressing of sesame oil, rice vinegar, ginger, and a hint of honey.

5. Mediterranean Chickpea Salad: A blend of chickpeas, cherry tomatoes, cucumber, red onion, feta cheese, and Kalamata olives, complemented by a dressing made with extra virgin olive oil, lemon juice, oregano, and a touch of garlic.

Remember to include a variety of colorful vegetables, healthy fats, and plant-based proteins to support hormone balance and overall well-being. Adjust the dressings according to your taste preferences and dietary needs. Enjoy your vibrant and hormone-balancing lunch!

Satisfying Grain Bowls

Satisfying grain bowls for hormone balance are nutrient-rich meals designed to support hormonal health. These bowls typically incorporate a balanced combination of whole grains, healthy fats, lean proteins, and a variety of colorful vegetables.

1. Whole Grains: Incorporating whole grains like quinoa, brown rice, or buckwheat provides complex carbohydrates that release energy slowly, helping to stabilize blood sugar levels and reduce insulin spikes. Stable blood sugar is essential for hormone balance.

2. Healthy Fats: Including sources of healthy fats like avocado, nuts, seeds, and olive oil supports hormone production and absorption. These fats also aid in reducing inflammation, which can positively impact hormone regulation.

3. Lean Proteins: Adding lean proteins such as grilled chicken, tofu, or legumes helps to maintain muscle mass and support hormone synthesis. Protein is essential for tissue repair and hormonal signaling.

4. Colorful Vegetables: A diverse array of vegetables provides essential vitamins, minerals, and antioxidants that aid in detoxification and promote hormone balance. Aim for a variety of colors to ensure a broad spectrum of nutrients.

5. Cruciferous Vegetables: Vegetables like broccoli, cauliflower, and kale contain compounds that support estrogen metabolism, helping to maintain a healthy balance of estrogen in the body.

6. Probiotic Foods: Fermented foods like sauerkraut, kimchi, or yogurt can promote a healthy gut microbiome, which plays a crucial role in hormone regulation.

7. Low-Glycemic Fruits: Opt for low-glycemic fruits like berries and cherries, which have less impact on blood sugar levels. These fruits are packed with antioxidants and can support hormone health.

8. Avoiding Processed Foods: Minimize processed and sugary foods, as they can disrupt hormone balance and lead to insulin resistance.

In summary, creating satisfying grain bowls for hormone balance involves a thoughtful combination of whole grains, healthy fats, lean proteins, colorful vegetables, and mindful food choices that promote overall hormonal health. By nourishing your body with these nutrient-dense ingredients, you can support hormone balance and overall well-being. For individualized nutritional guidance catered to your unique needs, don't forget to speak with a medical expert or a certified dietitian.

Hearty Soups and Stews

Hearty soups and stews are ideal for a satisfying lunch. They're comforting, nourishing, and can be prepared with a variety of ingredients. Here are some popular options:

1. Chicken Noodle Soup: This classic soup features tender chicken, vegetables, and egg noodles simmered in a flavorful broth. It's both comforting and nourishing, perfect for a chilly day.

2. Beef Stew: A hearty beef stew combines tender chunks of beef, potatoes, carrots, and other vegetables in a rich, savory broth. It's slow-cooked to perfection, resulting in tender meat and delicious flavors.

3. Vegetable Minestrone: Packed with a variety of vegetables, beans, and pasta,

minestrone is a wholesome option for vegetarians and vegans. The combination of flavors creates a hearty and nutrient-rich dish.

4. Lentil Soup: Lentils are a great source of protein and fiber, making lentil soup both filling and nutritious. It often includes vegetables and spices, providing a warm and satisfying lunch option.

5. Tomato Basil Soup: Creamy tomato soup infused with fresh basil is a classic favorite. It's simple yet delightful, especially when served with a grilled cheese sandwich.

6. Seafood Chowder: If you enjoy seafood, a hearty chowder with fish, shrimp, clams, or other seafood options might be your go-to choice. Creamy and flavorful, it's a delightful treat.

7. Spicy Chili: For those who crave bold flavors, a spicy chili with ground beef, beans, tomatoes, and chili spices is an excellent option. It's a crowd-pleaser and can be adjusted to your desired level of heat.

8. Potato Leek Soup: Creamy and velvety potato leek soup is a satisfying option for a light yet flavorful lunch. The

combination of potatoes and leeks creates a delicious taste.

When preparing hearty soups and stews, don't hesitate to customize the recipes to suit your preferences. They can be made in advance and reheated, making them a convenient and delicious lunch option. Enjoy!

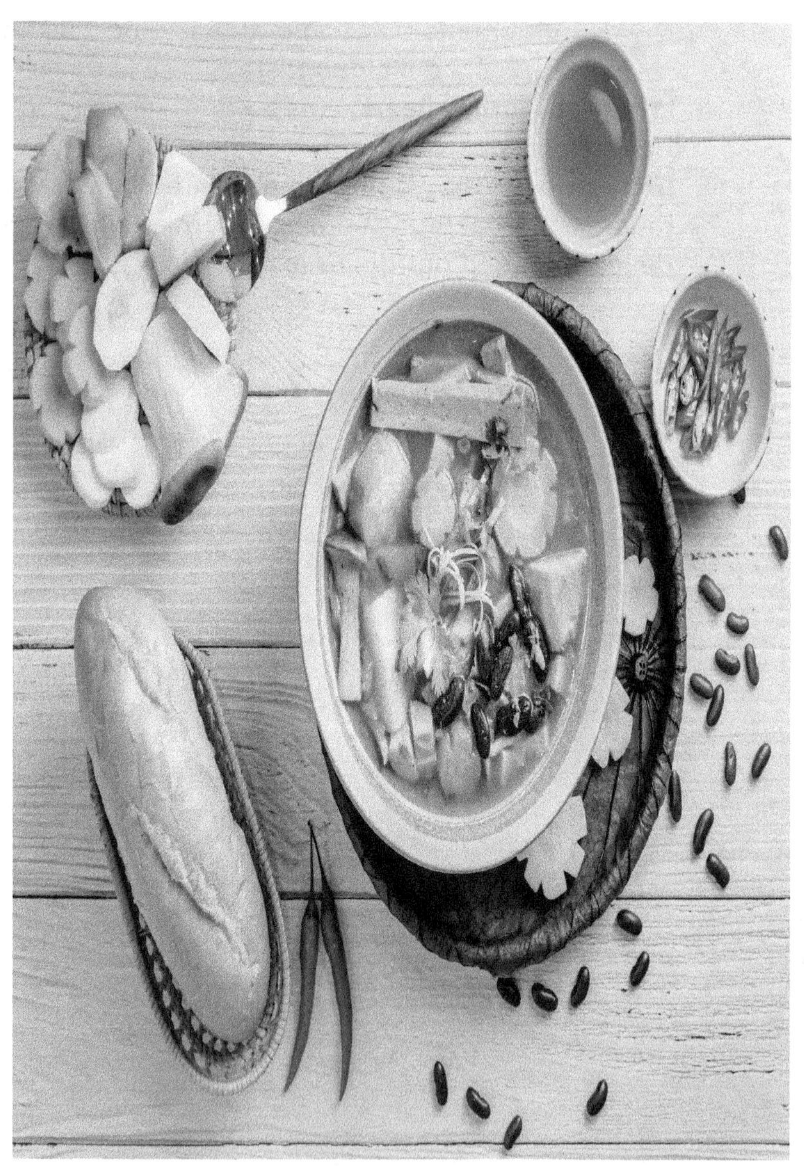

CHAPTER FIVE

Hormone-Friendly Dinner Options

Flavorful Plant-Based Dishes

Plant-based dishes can be incredibly flavorful and satisfying. Some popular options include:

1. Spicy Chickpea Curry: A delicious curry made with chickpeas, tomatoes, and aromatic spices.
2. Vegetable Stir-Fry: A colorful medley of fresh vegetables sautéed in a savory sauce.
3. Lentil Shepherd's Pie: A hearty pie filled with lentils, vegetables, and topped with creamy mashed potatoes.
4. Vegan Pad Thai: A zesty and tangy Thai noodle dish made with tofu, veggies, and a savory sauce.
5. Stuffed Bell Peppers: Bell peppers filled with quinoa, beans, and spices, then baked to perfection.

6. **Vegan Sushi Rolls:** Sushi rolls filled with avocado, cucumber, carrots, and other veggies.
7. **Eggplant Parmesan:** Breaded and baked eggplant slices topped with marinara sauce and vegan cheese.
8. **Mushroom Stroganoff:** A creamy and flavorful stroganoff made with mushrooms and plant-based sour cream.
9. **Jackfruit Tacos:** Shredded jackfruit cooked in smoky spices and served in taco shells with toppings.
10. **Mediterranean Chickpea Salad:** A refreshing salad with chickpeas, cucumbers, tomatoes, olives, and herbs, drizzled with a lemony dressing.

Remember, plant-based cuisine offers a wide variety of options to explore, from traditional dishes with a vegan twist to innovative creations bursting with flavor!

Protein-Packed Dinners

Protein-packed dinners are meals that contain a substantial amount of protein, which is essential for building and repairing tissues, supporting immune function, and maintaining overall health. Here are some examples of protein-packed dinners and their benefits:

Grilled Chicken with Quinoa and Roasted Vegetables:

1. Grilled chicken is a lean source of protein, while quinoa adds additional protein and is a complete source of essential amino acids. Roasted vegetables provide essential vitamins and minerals, making this meal well-rounded and nutritious.

Salmon with Sweet Potato and Asparagus:

2. Salmon is rich in omega-3 fatty acids and high-quality protein. Sweet potatoes are a great source of complex carbohydrates, and asparagus adds fiber and various vitamins to the meal.

Lentil and Chickpea Curry with Brown Rice:

3. Lentils and chickpeas are plant-based sources of protein and are also packed with fiber and essential nutrients. Brown rice complements this dish by providing additional protein and complex carbohydrates.

Tofu Stir-Fry with Broccoli and Cashews:

4. Tofu is an excellent plant-based protein source with a versatile texture. Broccoli adds essential vitamins, while cashews provide healthy fats and a satisfying crunch to the dish.

Beef and Vegetable Skewers with Quinoa Salad:

5. Lean beef provides high-quality protein and important minerals like iron and zinc. Vegetable skewers add color and nutrients, and a quinoa salad complements the meal with more protein and fiber.

Including protein-packed dinners in your diet can help you feel fuller, maintain muscle mass, and support your overall well-being. Remember to balance your meals with other nutrients, such as healthy fats, carbohydrates, and a variety of fruits and vegetables.

Healthy Stir-Fries and Sauteed Delicacies

Healthy stir-fries and sauteed delicacies are flavorful and nutritious dishes that can be easily prepared with a variety of ingredients.

These cooking methods involve quick cooking over high heat, which helps retain the natural flavors and nutrients of the ingredients. Here are some tips for making healthy stir-fries and sautéed delicacies:

1. **Choose Lean Proteins:** Opt for lean protein sources like chicken breast, turkey, tofu, or shrimp. These proteins are lower in saturated fats and can be cooked quickly, preserving their tenderness.

2. **Load Up on Veggies:** Include an array of colorful vegetables such as broccoli, bell peppers, carrots, snap peas, and zucchini. Veggies provide essential vitamins, minerals, and fiber, enhancing the overall nutritional value of the dish.

3. **Healthy Fats:** Use heart-healthy fats like olive oil, avocado oil, or coconut oil for sautéing. These fats add richness to the dish while promoting good cholesterol levels.

4. **Flavorful Sauces:** Make your own sauces with reduced-sodium soy sauce, ginger, garlic, and a touch of honey or maple syrup for natural sweetness. Avoid store-bought sauces with excessive added sugars and preservatives.

5. **Mindful Seasonings:** Experiment with herbs and spices to enhance the taste without relying on excessive salt. Fresh herbs like basil, cilantro, or parsley add a burst of freshness.

6. **Nourishing Grains:** If you wish to add grains, opt for whole grains like quinoa, brown rice, or whole wheat noodles, which provide more fiber and nutrients compared to refined grains.

7. **Controlled Cooking Time:** Stir-frying and sautéing are quick methods, so be cautious not to overcook the vegetables to preserve their crunchiness and nutrients.

Now, let's differentiate between stir-frying and sauteing:

- **Stir-frying:** This method involves cooking small pieces of ingredients, such as meat and vegetables, in a hot wok or skillet with minimal oil, stirring them constantly. The high heat ensures that the food cooks quickly and retains its texture and flavor.

- **Sauteing:** In sauteing, ingredients are cooked in a shallow pan over medium-high heat with a small amount of oil. The ingredients are tossed or stirred occasionally until they are tender and lightly browned.

Both stir-frying and sauteing are excellent techniques for creating healthy, tasty dishes that showcase the natural flavors of the ingredients. They are versatile cooking methods that allow you to experiment with various ingredients while maintaining their nutritional integrity. Enjoy your delicious and nutritious stir-fries and sauteed delicacies!

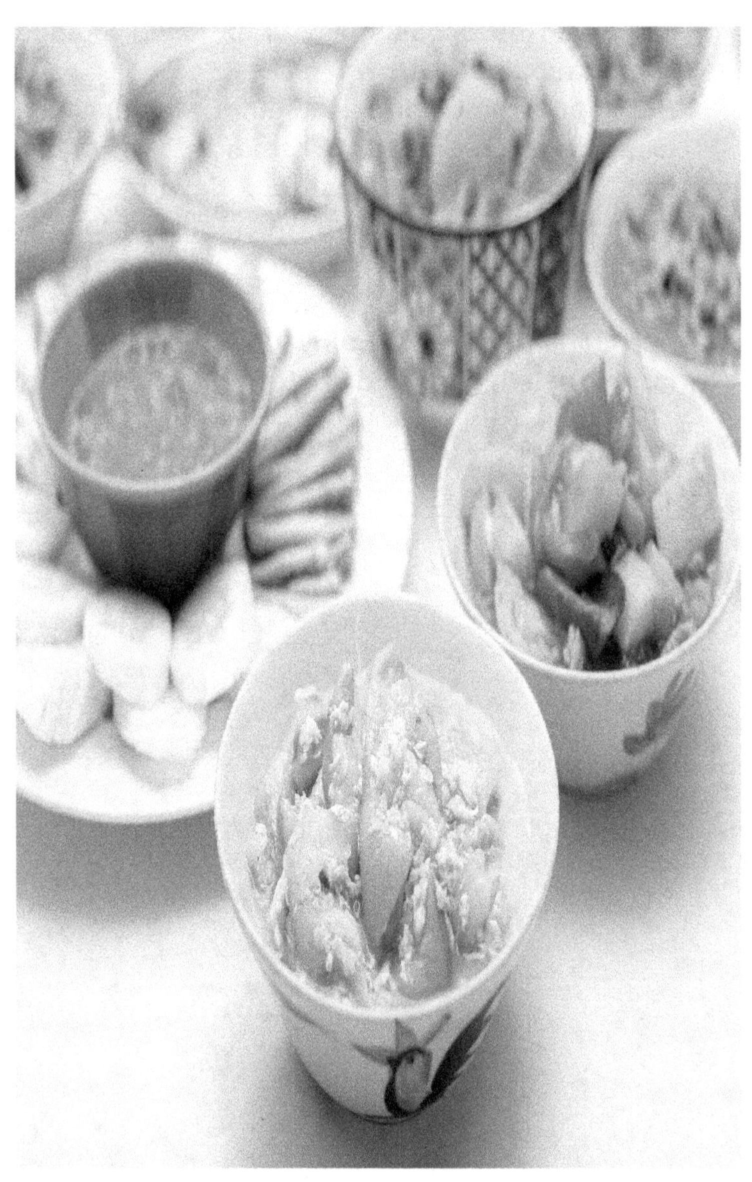

CHAPTER SIX

Snacks to Support Hormonal Equilibrium

Guilt-Free Energy Bites

Guilt-Free Energy Bites are nutritious and delicious snacks that are designed to provide a boost of energy without the guilt of consuming unhealthy ingredients. They are often made with natural, whole-food ingredients that offer a balance of carbohydrates, protein, and healthy fats.

Here's a simple recipe for Guilt-Free Energy Bites:

Ingredients:

- 1 cup rolled oats (gluten-free if needed)
- 1/2 cup nut butter (e.g., almond butter, peanut butter)
- A sweetness-enhancing 1/3 cup of honey or maple syrup
- 1 /2 cup ground flaxseed
- 1/2 cup shredded coconut (unsweetened)
- Cacao nibs or half a cup of dark chocolate chips
- 1 teaspoon vanilla extract

- A pinch of salt

Instructions:

1. In a large mixing bowl, combine rolled oats, nut butter, honey (or maple syrup), ground flaxseed, shredded coconut, dark chocolate chips, vanilla extract, and a pinch of salt.
2. You can add a bit additional nut butter or honey/maple syrup if the mixture seems too dry.
3. Once the mixture is well mixed, cover the bowl and refrigerate for about 30 minutes to make it easier to handle.
4. After refrigerating, take small portions of the mixture and roll them into bite-sized balls using your hands.
5. Place the energy bites on a baking sheet lined with parchment paper and refrigerate for another 30 minutes to firm them up.
6. Once the energy bites are firm, transfer them to an airtight container and store them in the refrigerator for up to one week.

Now, let me explain why these Energy Bites are considered guilt-free:

1. Nutritious Ingredients: These energy bites are made with whole-food

ingredients like oats, nut butter, ground flaxseed, and shredded coconut, which provide a good balance of complex carbohydrates, healthy fats, and fiber. These nutrients help sustain energy levels and keep you feeling fuller for longer.

2. No Refined Sugars: Instead of using refined sugars, these bites are sweetened naturally with honey or maple syrup, which are better alternatives that won't cause rapid spikes in blood sugar levels.

3. Protein-Rich: The nut butter and flaxseed in the recipe add protein content, which is essential for muscle repair and maintenance, as well as keeping you feeling satisfied.

4. Good Fats: The nut butter and shredded coconut are sources of healthy fats, which are beneficial for brain health and maintaining overall well-being.

5. Convenient and Portable: Guilt-Free Energy Bites are easy to make and can be stored in the refrigerator for quick and on-the-go snacks, perfect for busy days or as a pre- or post-workout treat.

Remember, while these energy bites are a healthier alternative to many store-bought snacks, portion control is still important. Moderation is key to enjoying guilt-free indulgences!

Wholesome Trail Mixes

Wholesome trail mixes are nutritious and energy-packed snacks made from a mix of various dried fruits, nuts, seeds, and sometimes other ingredients like dark chocolate or coconut flakes. They are a popular choice for hikers, outdoor enthusiasts, and health-conscious individuals due to their portability, convenience, and balanced nutritional content.

The typical ingredients found in a wholesome trail mix include:

1. Nuts: Almonds, walnuts, cashews, or peanuts provide healthy fats, protein, and essential minerals like magnesium and zinc.
2. Dried Fruits: Raisins, cranberries, apricots, or dates add natural sweetness and supply vitamins, fiber, and antioxidants.
3. Seeds: Sunflower seeds, pumpkin seeds, or chia seeds contribute to the mix's nutritional value by offering protein,

healthy fats, and essential micronutrients.

4. Dark Chocolate: In moderation, dark chocolate chips can be added for a delightful touch while providing antioxidants and potentially mood-enhancing properties.
5. Coconut Flakes: These provide a tropical twist and offer healthy fats and dietary fiber.

The benefits of wholesome trail mixes lie in their nutrient-dense composition, which can boost energy levels, support heart health, and aid in weight management. They offer a combination of carbohydrates, proteins, and fats, providing a sustained source of energy during physical activities or as a quick pick-me-up throughout the day.

Moreover, trail mixes are typically free from artificial additives, preservatives, and excess sugars often found in conventional snacks, making them a healthier alternative. However, it's essential to be mindful of portion sizes, as trail mixes can be calorie-dense.

Wholesome trail mixes are easy to customize based on individual preferences and dietary needs. Whether you're seeking an energy boost during a hike or a satisfying and nutritious snack on the go, these mixes can be a delightful and healthy choice. Remember to check ingredient labels if you're purchasing pre-packaged trail mixes to ensure they align with your health goals.

Hormone-Balancing Dip and Veggie Sticks

Here's a recipe for a Hormone-Balancing Dip and Veggie Sticks, along with an explanation of how it can potentially support hormone balance:

Ingredients for the Hormone-Balancing Dip:

- 1 cup plain Greek yogurt
- 1 tablespoon tahini
- 1 tablespoon fresh lemon juice
- 1 clove garlic, minced
- 1 teaspoon ground flaxseed
- 1 teaspoon ground turmeric
- 1/2 teaspoon ground cinnamon
- Salt and pepper to taste

Ingredients for Veggie Sticks:

- Carrot sticks
- Cucumber sticks
- Celery sticks
- Bell pepper strips
- Broccoli florets

Instructions:

1. In a mixing bowl, combine the Greek yogurt, tahini, lemon juice, minced garlic, ground flaxseed, ground turmeric, ground cinnamon, salt, and pepper. Mix everything until well combined.
2. Taste the dip and adjust the seasoning if needed, according to your preferences.
3. Wash and cut the vegetables into sticks or strips for easy dipping.
4. Serve the Hormone-Balancing Dip with the Veggie Sticks, and enjoy!

Explanation of Hormone-Balancing Properties:

This dip contains several ingredients that are believed to support hormone balance:

1. Greek yogurt: It is a good source of protein and calcium, which are essential for hormone production and function.
2. Tahini: Rich in healthy fats, tahini can support hormone regulation and overall hormonal health.
3. Lemon juice: Lemon is a good source of vitamin C, which helps in hormone synthesis and supports the immune system.
4. Flaxseed: Flaxseed contains lignans, which are phytoestrogens that may help balance estrogen levels in the body.

5. Turmeric: Known for its anti-inflammatory properties, turmeric can help reduce inflammation, which may positively impact hormone balance.
6. Cinnamon: Cinnamon can help improve insulin sensitivity, which is important for maintaining balanced blood sugar levels and hormone regulation.
7. Garlic: Garlic contains sulfur compounds that can support liver function, helping the body metabolize and balance hormones.

Including a variety of colorful veggies like carrots, cucumbers, celery, bell peppers, and broccoli in the Veggie Sticks provides essential vitamins, minerals, and antioxidants that contribute to overall health and hormonal well-being.

It's important to note that while these ingredients may offer potential hormonal benefits, individual responses can vary, and dietary choices should be personalized based on specific health needs and goals. As always, consulting with a healthcare professional or a registered dietitian can provide personalized guidance for your hormone-balancing needs.

CHAPTER SEVEN

Desserts for Hormone Harmony

Sweet Treats with Natural Sweeteners

Sweet treats with natural sweeteners are a delicious and healthier alternative to desserts made with refined sugars. Natural sweeteners are derived from plants and provide sweetness without the negative impacts associated with processed sugars. Some popular natural sweeteners include honey, maple syrup, agave nectar, and coconut sugar.

When making sweet treats with natural sweeteners, you can easily substitute them for refined sugars in recipes like cookies, cakes, and puddings. They not only add sweetness but also contribute unique flavors and additional nutrients.

Honey, for example, contains antioxidants and has antimicrobial properties. Minerals like zinc and manganese are abundant in maple syrup. Agave nectar is ideal for people controlling their blood sugar levels because of its low glycemic index. Coconut sugar contains small amounts of vitamins and minerals like potassium and iron.

However, it's essential to remember that natural sweeteners, while healthier, still contain calories and should be consumed in moderation. They can also impact the texture and moisture of baked goods, so some recipe adjustments may be necessary.

When enjoying sweet treats made with natural sweeteners, savor them in moderation as part of a balanced diet. If you have particular dietary concerns or medical issues, always seek the advice of a healthcare.

Indulgent yet Healthy Dessert Creations

Indulgent yet healthy dessert creations focus on satisfying your sweet cravings while incorporating nutritious ingredients. Here are some examples and explanations:

1. Avocado Chocolate Mousse: Avocado provides a creamy texture without using heavy cream, and it's packed with healthy fats and fiber.
2. Banana Nice Cream: Blend frozen bananas for a dairy-free ice cream

alternative, rich in potassium and natural sweetness.

3. **Chia Seed Pudding:** Chia seeds soaked in milk or plant-based milk create a pudding-like consistency rich in omega-3 fatty acids and fiber.

4. **Greek Yogurt Parfait:** Layer Greek yogurt with fresh fruits, nuts, and a drizzle of honey for a protein-packed and calcium-rich treat.

5. **Dark Chocolate-Covered Berries:** Dip antioxidant-rich berries like strawberries, blueberries, or raspberries in melted dark chocolate for a decadent yet heart-healthy dessert.

6. **Baked Apple Crisp:** Use oats, cinnamon, and a touch of honey to create a crunchy topping for baked apples, a delightful source of vitamins and fiber.

7. **Coconut Bliss Balls:** Combine shredded coconut, nuts, and dates into bite-sized balls, offering a natural sweetness and healthy fats.

8. **Almond Butter Brownies:** Swap traditional butter for almond butter in your brownie recipe for added protein and monounsaturated fats.

9. Fruit Sorbet: Blend frozen fruits like mango, pineapple, or mixed berries for a refreshing, low-calorie dessert option.
10. Quinoa Chocolate Chip Cookies: Incorporate quinoa flour and dark chocolate chips into your cookie recipe for added protein and a boost of antioxidants.

These indulgent yet healthy dessert creations prioritize nutrient-dense ingredients and limit refined sugars, unhealthy fats, and artificial additives. They provide a guilt-free way to enjoy sweet treats while supporting your overall well-being. Just keep in mind to consume them in moderation as part of a healthy diet.

Meal Planning Tips for Hormonal Wellness

Here are some meal planning tips for hormonal wellness:

1. Balance Macronutrients: Include a mix of healthy fats, proteins, and complex carbohydrates in each meal to help stabilize blood sugar levels and support hormone production.

2. **Choose Whole Foods:** Opt for whole, unprocessed foods like fruits, vegetables, whole grains, and lean proteins to provide essential nutrients for hormonal balance.
3. **Prioritize Omega-3s:** Incorporate foods rich in omega-3 fatty acids, such as salmon, chia seeds, and flaxseeds, which can help reduce inflammation and support hormone regulation.
4. **Limit Added Sugars:** Minimize consumption of sugary foods and drinks as they can lead to insulin spikes and hormonal imbalances.
5. **Include Phytoestrogen-Rich Foods:** Foods like soy, lentils, and flaxseeds contain natural plant compounds that can help regulate estrogen levels.
6. **Support Gut Health:** Include fermented foods like yogurt, sauerkraut, and kefir to promote a healthy gut microbiome, which plays a role in hormonal regulation.
7. **Stay Hydrated:** Drink plenty of water throughout the day to support overall health and hormonal balance.
8. **Mindful Eating:** Pay attention to hunger cues and practice mindful eating to

prevent overeating and support digestion.

9. Limit Caffeine and Alcohol: Excessive caffeine and alcohol intake can disrupt hormonal balance, so consume them in moderation.

10. Manage Stress: High stress levels can impact hormone production. Spend time in nature or practice stress-relieving exercises like yoga or meditation.

Remember, individual needs may vary, so it's always a good idea to consult with a healthcare professional or registered dietitian for personalized meal planning advice.

CHAPTER EIGHT

Conclusion

In conclusion, the Hormone Harmony cookbook offers a comprehensive and valuable resource for individuals seeking to improve their hormonal health naturally. By providing a diverse range of nutritious and hormone-balancing recipes, this guide promotes overall well-being and addresses specific hormonal issues effectively. Emphasizing the importance of balanced nutrition and mindful eating, it empowers readers to take control of their hormonal health. Incorporating these recipes into one's daily routine can lead to positive outcomes and a healthier, more balanced life. Always seek the advice and direction of a qualified healthcare practitioner when making decisions about your hormone health.

www.ingramcontent.com/pod-product-compliance
Lightning Source LLC
Chambersburg PA
CBHW071118260726
48661CB00006B/2643